I0420445

Disclaimer:

I am a Health Coach who received my training from the Institute of Integrative Nutrition in New York, NY, USA. I have studied over 100 dietary theories, practical lifestyle management techniques, and innovative coaching methods with some of the world's top health and wellness experts, including Dr. Andrew Weil, Dr. Deepak Chopra, Dr. David Katz, Dr. Walter Willett, Dr. Mark Hyman, Dr. Alejandro Junger, Dr. John Douillard, Dr. Liz Lipski, Dr. Josh Axe, Donna Gates, and many other leading researchers and nutrition authorities. Furthermore, I also hold a Master of Science in Biotechnology with specialty in Immunology.

However, I am not a medical doctor, dietician, nor nutritionist. I do not hold a degree in medicine, dietetics, or nutrition. I make no claims to any specialized medical training, nor do I give medical advice or prescriptions. This content is not intended to diagnose, treat or cure any disease. It is intended to be provided for informational, educational, and self- empowerment purposes ONLY. Please consult with your doctor or wellness team if you have any questions regarding this book, and then make your own well-informed decisions based upon what is best for your unique genetics, culture, conditions, and stage of life.

All content within this book is based on my personal knowledge, opinions, and experience as a holistic health coach. Please consult a medical advisor regarding medications or medical advice.

I look forward to helping you create a life with Endless Energy.

Dedication:

This book is dedicated to everyone that suffers from low energy and feels as if they are barely surviving in their day to day life. With these 6 simple steps you can increase your quality of life, health and happiness, and achieve a THRIVING existence. You have the power within you to make this life everything you have ever dreamt about, so start NOW. I am here to guide you.

Acknowledgement:

To the doctor that thought I was depressed and mentally ill, if it had not been for him, I would not have looked into the concept of using FOOD AS MEDICINE.

To my mom and dad for always encouraging me to do my best and do what I love. Thanks to all of you for making this dream a reality!

To my brother for being my spiritual guide and leading me into this path of transcendence and personal growth!

Of course to my loving husband, who has been a great support through sickness, through healing, and now through building my Awesome Healthy Life. I would not be where I am today, as a healthy entrepreneur, if it were not for his support and love! You are the love of my life, Mads Berge-Lind.

Table of Content:

My Story

My name is Linda Berge-Lind. I am half-Norwegian and half-Icelandic, but I grew up and have lived most of my life in Denmark.

I earned a Master of Science in Biotechnology with a specialty in Immunology and normally a person with this education works in the medical industry, either making prescription drugs or doing research. So how did I end up as a Health Coach?

Five years ago, after a spring full of vaccines, yeast medication and antibiotics, my health began to deteriorate. Over the next two year symptoms kept sneaking up on me, and at the end of year 2, I had more than 30 different symptoms. Some symptoms were physical and other symptoms were mental; it was everything from joint and muscle pain to stomach bloating. I suffered from memory loss and depression, and felt completely fatigued. At the point when things were at their worst, I was isolated and lonely. I had no energy and at times I actually went to the restroom or the locker room while at work to take naps, just to try and get through the day. It was really, really tough. When talking with people, I often asked the same questions repeatedly because I did not remember asking them. These forgotten conversations embarrassed me.

It took me a while to realize that it was not normal to have so many symptoms, and when I

finally saw a doctor and said, "I have all these symptoms and I don't know what's wrong. I just need to get well." The doctor looked me in the eye and told me, "Linda, there's nothing medically wrong with you. It's all in your head." I left that day feeling defeated and thought, "Could I really be mentally sick? What's going on?"

So there I was: 28 years old, unable to bike or exercise because of the pain, too embarrassed to see friends because I could not hold a conversation, and with no passion for life. I was in survival mode.

I could not give up on my life so I decided to do what my education and training taught me: I researched! Not for the newest cancer cure or prescription medicine, but for a way to find the treatment for my own sufferings. I needed to fight and knew there had to be a solution somewhere. I studied everything I could about how to get well. I read scientific articles, different self-help books, blogs, and so on. Given my poor short term memory, this was hard work and required all the effort I could muster. In the end, the solution started to dawn on me: FOOD AS MEDICINE. Many people with the same symptoms posted online that they felt better by changing their diet, so I thought, that's the way I need to go.

I undertook a journey of trying everything that everyone else tried. I attempted the Candida Diet, I went gluten-free, removed all sugars from my diet, and then all grains and milk as well. I tried everything backwards and forwards, and I almost always felt better with each new diet. However, I was still fatigued, and I still had some problems that would not go away. Even though I felt better, none of the solutions I tested worked consistently. At this point I needed to do something different so I started using what I today call the Awareness Journal. I wrote down what I ate and how I felt during the day; I documented anything in the environment that affected me. Shortly after starting the Awareness Journal I decided to try to remove all

the food triggers that I read about, but instead of removing them individually, I removed all of them at the same time

Doing these two things, taking high quality probiotics, eating easy digestible and nutrients-

dense wholefoods, and implementing simple lifestyle changes I cured myself within 3 months. I am so thankful that I did not give up on myself, and today I can proudly state that I am still 100% free of any symptoms and have been for the last 3 years. I am living the life of my dreams: I wake up every morning fully rested and happy to get out of bed and on with my day.

After I healed my body, I knew I could not go back to my old job in the medical industry. I had a more important message to tell people, use FOOD AS MEDICINE, and achieve a healthy life with vibrant energy. I decided to become a Health Coach from the Institute for Integrative Nutrition. Today I am the CEO and founder of Awesome Healthy Life, and I promote health and happiness all over the world.

After seeing how easy and how massive an impact it can have on people's lives when done right, I became passionate about sharing my hard earned knowledge with the world. I have taken everything I learned from my studies and trial and error process and put all the key learnings in to The 6 Simple Steps to fast track you past all the unnecessary and ineffective FAD diets and directly to the lifestyle that will give you Endless Energy, and take you from just surviving to THRIVING.

Benefits of The 6 Simple Steps

My mission in life is to inspire YOU to take charge of your own life and create a wonderful healthy life full of energy and joy. I have made the process much simpler for you so you can skip the trial and error I needed to go though. Follow the 6 simple steps in this book, and you will take your life to the next level.

What would you say if I told you that you could stop just simply surviving day to day and start living a life full of energy and purpose? There is no more need for a daily dose of caffeine to keep you going; you will wake up rejuvenated and ready to have fantastic day, to be present in every moment. With this book, you have the simple and exact steps you need in order to increase your energy levels, maintain a stable and happy mood, and reclaim your passion for life. You can create the life of your dreams.

As a part of Endless Energy, from surviving to THRIVING, I will guide you through each and every step ensuring that you can follow through. Before we go through the steps, the benefits of success are:

- Increased energy all through the day
- Balanced blood sugar → lower risk of diabetes
- Healthier and more vibrant life
- Improved digestion
- Reduced allergy
- Weight loss
- Reduced inflammation
- Reduce addictions to caffeine, sugar and processed foods
- Hormonal balance
- Less muscle and joint pain
- Free of fatigue

- Better sleep, more rested

- Happier with an elevated and stable mood

- Improved immune system

A client of mine suffered from unclear thinking and stress for a long period of time. She did not feel fully present with her children or husband. Work problems plagued her and followed her home. That completely changed after she completed the 6 steps. She learned basic tools in order to be more present with her family and gained valuable knowledge to better handle stressful situations.

Rather than worry about dinner or focus on being tired, she changed her way of thinking and used her new tools to come up with new ideas. For example, "why not have a picnic at the playground for dinner?" So she did and her family not only enjoyed eating outdoors, but they loved the quality time together as a family. She quickly noticed that her children were happier because with the help of these 6 simple steps, they were aware that their mom was fully present in their daily lives.

The same way these steps changed my client's life, they can also change your life for the better. Some clients report back to me that they feel the difference in just one week, and it just keeps getting better and better! They have more energy and are calmer and more focused in their daily activities. They experience a sense of being more present in every moment, and are therefore more productive at work. And when they get home from work, they are better able to focus on their families and friends making for richer, more memorable quality time.

Another one of my clients came to me with constipation issues, and after only one week of implementing half of the steps she called me to tell me she had experienced what I call "one- minute elimination"; in and out of the restroom in one minute. This was a new experience for her and allowed her to remove toxins that were draining her and affecting her daily life from her body easier and faster. It has increased her health and wellness and she now lives a happier, fuller life with much more energy. She also stated that I saved her a tremendous amount of time that was previously spent reading magazines while using the restroom.

When you follow the steps to increase your energy level and gain a bigger quality of life, you tend to think bigger. The possibilities for where you can take your life, with your good thoughts and feelings, are endless. Two of my clients recently decided to start their own businesses because they gained the energy, focus and passion to do it. Before using the simple steps, it was just a thought with no action. It is amazing and I feel honoured to experience my clients' expression of themselves and their belief in possibilities. Before, it was just a dream, but now, they are making it a reality.

When having optimum health and being more energized, the things you can do with your life suddenly become clearer. If you did not lack the energy what would you be doing right now? What are your dreams? What is your passion?

My experience is that people who go through these 6 steps re-claim their passion for life, and so much more. They increase their energy are reminded that the possibilities are endless. So, what are your dreams?

How to Succeed with The 6 simple Steps

A lot of people all over the world feel like they are merely surviving in their daily life. Life goes past so fast and people forget to enjoy their moments. We are busy people that have ambitions and want to experience everything, but often forget to take care of ourselves. When we do not take care of ourselves over a long period of time, and add in the fast solutions for food, caffeine and less sleep, our bodies become drained and fatigue sets in.

A poor life balance is very important to focus on because if we ignore that balance, we will continue in the same pattern as we have done for years and nothing will change! Furthermore, we will teach our children bad habits and show them that this is how life is, this is how we are supposed to live. Our bad habits will be passed down through generations. What children observe until the age of 6 become their own "programs", by which they will live their life.

With these simple steps you will not only see the benefits in your own life right here and now, but you will also teach your children to live a more balanced, centred and happy life.

When I introduce people to the steps, a lot of them are very sceptical and believe them to be unmanageable. But after a short coaching session people are ready to take action. Ask yourself the following questions:

- What will your life be like in 3 years if you continue feeling fatigued?
- How are other people influenced by your lack of change?
- How are you affected if you do not change anything?
- How will others be influenced by your boundless energy?
- What will it feel like when you achieve your goals?
- How will other people be affected when you get Endless Energy?

- Why are you afraid of change?

- What is the worst possible thing that could happen if you did the 6 simple steps?

- Is that worst possible thing really going to happen? – and if it does, what is worse, that or dying with regret?

- If these fears are not as bad as you thought they were, or you realize that the regret is just as bad, what are 2 things you would start doing now?

Find out what motivates you to have Endless Energy, and improve your quality of life, health and happiness. We are all unique and have different reasons for why we want a specific thing. What do you feel is missing in your life? What passions and emotions are you searching for? These passions and emotions are the key to your success; focus on them while you ask yourself the above questions. With your goals and intentions clear in your mind throughout your day, it is easier to actually follow through and focus on what is needed for you to succeed in reaching your goals and to have the life you really want for yourself. Some people are motivated by the fear of what will happen if they do not change while others are motivated by the positive things that will happen if they follow through. What motivates you?

After coaching my clients on the topic of fear and resistance, they normally just jump right into it and start doing the steps that are needed. A lot of them actually say that their way of thinking has changed, and they cannot understand why they saw it as a problem before the coaching session.

Step #1: Awareness for Endless Energy

Create awareness in your life! We are all unique individuals and we all react different to the environment we are in and the food we eat. Please take an extra look at your own life and understand what makes your body thrive. Are there any connections between what you eat and how you feel? Does certain food trigger a change in mood and/or symptoms? If there are triggers, I encourage you to remove the triggers that leave you feeling low and fatigued.

Some of the foods you notice that do not work for you might be considered healthy, but listen to your body, it knows what is best for you. I had this issue myself. There is a connection between eating almonds and pain in my left shoulder. I know almonds are healthy and while today I can tolerate almonds very well, at a point in my life I reacted negatively towards them. It is also important to know that during our lifetimes, our bodies change. What was good for us five years ago may not be good for us today. It all depends on where we are in life, the environment we are in, and our general health.

To put this awareness into a manageable structure for you, I have created a template for an awareness journal. See the template at the end of this section.

Pay attention not only to food but also other aspects of your life. Some years ago, I always felt really sick in the morning, and I connected it to my job. I believed that I needed an excuse like, "Oh, my stomach hurts. Maybe I should stay home." I figured out that it was my stressful work environment that did not resonate with who I am as a person. In the end I quit my job. This is probably not the right solution for most people, but if you find that your job is draining you, I encourage you to take action. Find something within your job that you like and try to do more of that, and try to reduce the things that irritate you or cause you stress. Another thing you can do is to speak with your boss about how to make your day more enjoyable. The more you like your job, the better you are at it, which in the long run gives you more energy and better results! In other words, every bosses dream!

It is also good to have awareness about other situations in your life that leaves you with an unpleasant feeling or makes you tired. Malls for example has a lot of toxins and high stress levels from the crowds, so maybe you are fatigued after shopping trip.

Look at your life and ask yourself: Are there any persons or situations that drain your energy? What is it that gives you energy and what is it that drains you? Keep this kind of focus throughout your day, week and life. When you do identify things, persons or situations that rob your energy, investigate what you can do to change the situation. Is the situation really that bad, is it because you are having focus on all the negative aspects (See Positive Thinking for Endless Energy), or do you need to take some kind of action to achieve more energy?

A friend of mine had problems with constipation, and added a lot of fibre supplements to her diet. She felt that the fibre only made the problem worse, but whenever she talked to people about it, they told her she was being stupid because fibres are healthy and support good digestion. When she shared her story with me, I told her that fibres are not always good, and there are some people with gut problems where fibres actually make them feel worse. She felt so relieved when I said that, because what she was experiencing finally made sense to her. What I am trying to say with this story is that we all need to learn from and trust our body's signals. It really does know what is best for us.

Even though, I do not use the Awareness Journal on a regular basis anymore, I still keep this awareness in my life. Whenever I do not feel completely healthy, or when I feel out of balance in some way, the first thing I ask myself is: What happened the last couple of weeks and am I eating something that could trigger these issues?

How to use The Awareness Journal

1. Write down the time of your meal or when you notice a mood or symptom change.

2. Write down everything you eat and drink immediately after eating or drinking.

3. Note where and what you are doing while eating.

4. How did you feel during or right after eating?

5. How did you feel 2 hours after eating?

6. Write down any difference in mood, feelings or physical symptoms throughout the day.

7. When you do feel a change? Take note of what you did right before the change.

When you write down what you are eating it is important not to generalize. Do not write Burger, but be more specific. 100% beef meat with cucumber, tomato, Heinz mayonnaise and ketchup on a whole-wheat (store-bought) burger bun. Always include sauces and gravies. Do not forget to write down "extras," such as soda, salad dressing, butter, sour cream, sugar, salt, pepper. It is important to have as many details as possible, otherwise it will be hard to be a detective in your own life. How much you eat of a certain food is not as important, since we are not counting calories, but it is important to notice if you did eat too much.

Write down where you eat and what you do while you eat since this can also influence how you feel after your meal. If you eat a healthy lunch in a cafeteria that is busy, you might still get an upset stomach with bloating simply from the stress of not having a quiet moment while you eat. You might eat too fast and forget to chew your food because you are in a hurry. Write what room or part of the house you are in when you eat. Take note if you eat in a restaurant, fast-food chain or your car. All notes count! Also mention if you are driving, watching TV, working, chatting on the phone, having a nice family dinner or whatever you are doing. This can also be used to be more aware of situations like the one I described where I did not want to go to work. My location was at home and the action was getting ready for work and the symptom were often nausea and stomach aches.

When paying attention to how you feel after eating and throughout the day, you can look for these suggestions:

Physical changes:

Gas, belly bloating, insomnia, lack in/better concentration, muscle/joint pain, cramps, muscle weakness, left you hungry, left you wanting something more, got a sweet tooth, increase/decrease in energy, brain fog, memory loss, fatigue, coughing, restlessness, breathing pattern, increase/decrease in focus, alertness, exhaustion.

Emotional changes:

Sad, mad, anxious, bored, depressed, scattered, irritable, hyper, anxious, panic attack, confident, excited, energized, happy, interested, focused, calm, relaxed, patient.

Keep your journal with you all day and write down everything you eat or drink. A piece of chocolate, a handful of almonds, a can of soda or some candy. Everything can change how you feel and leave you fatigued, so be honest with yourself. It is your life and you have the power to make it a better one today! Do not depend on your memory at the end of the day.

Use the Awareness Journal below to write down what you eat and how you feel after each meal, as well as other triggers you experience in your life. Are you energized or exhausted? Do you notice any triggers that leave you fatigued? Think of it like this: You are a scientist and observer in your own life, and you are looking for hidden links within your journal. Pay attention to that which gives you energy and that which takes away energy. By gathering this information systematically over a couple of weeks or longer it will give you a much more objective and detailed view than simply relying on memory.

The Awareness Journal Template

TIME	Place/Action	Food	Mood & possible Symptoms

Step #2: Food for Endless Energy

Step #1: Awareness of Endless Energy teaches you how to pay attention to what gives you energy and what drains you of your energy.

As an extension of this step, there are some food groups that often trigger fatigue. I encourage you to try and remove them for a minimum period of 2 weeks to see how they affect your daily life.

I will introduce you to a few simple ways to eat that which will improve your health and leave you with endless energy.

Remove Foods that Trigger Symptoms and Fatigue

The five foods that often trigger symptoms and leave people fatigued are sugar, processed foods, grains, legumes and dairy. Below I give a short introduction to why this is so, and why I encourage you to try a life without them.

I want to emphasize that removing all five triggers at the same time will give you the best results. If you do decide to add the foods back in after removing them for a long period of time, you should do so by adding in one thing at a time and pay close attention to your Awareness Journal to determine if there is any shift in how you feel either physically or emotionally.

Sugar

The average American person consumes 152 lbs. (69 kg) sugar per year, much of which is hidden in processed foods. The body cannot tolerate this large amount of refined sugar, and it can be very damaging to vital organs in the body.

Sugar, which is a mix of short-chained, soluble carbohydrates like glycose and fructose, contains no fiber, no minerals, no protein, no enzymes, no fat and is empty calories void of any vital nutrients. When digesting sugar, the body needs to borrow nutrients from the healthy cells to be able to complete the metabolism. In order to use the energy in the sugar, the body is stripped of important nutrients like calcium, sodium, potassium and magnesium and also various vitamins and enzymes. High sugar consumption over a long period will deplete the body, and high amounts of minerals and vitamins are needed to correct the imbalance.

High amounts of sugar leaves your body weakened which affects the organ cells and prevents the immune system from functioning optimally. A weakened immune system can lead to yeast infections, poor digestion, skin rashes, joint pain, diabetes, liver problems, headaches, poor sleep, bad breath, cravings, disease, and poor concentration.

Apart from leaving your body depleted of vital nutrients, sugar is also known to elevate the blood sugar or glucose levels. When pure table sugar hits your bloodstream, your blood sugar increases way to high, and as a result, the body produces insulin to lower the glucose levels.

What often happens is that the body produces too much insulin (to combat the excessively high blood sugar level) and afterwards the glucose levels drop too low, resulting in a crashing feeling after the spike. If this continues for an extended period, your body can become resistant to the insulin. This means that the receptors on the cells do not recognize insulin as well as before and the production of insulin goes up. Over time, people become more and more insulin resistant and they end up having elevated levels of insulin and high blood sugar. Both are related to several diseases such as type 2 diabetes, cardiovascular diseases, obesity, increased risk of cancer, hormonal unbalances and lowered fertility. Maybe you are not the person that ends up with any of these diagnoses, but one thing is sure, eating sugar drains your body from vital nutrients and contributes to your feelings of low energy. Give it a try and remove sugar from your diet for 2 weeks, and see how you feel.

Depending on your current level of sugar intake, withdraw from sugar might result in cravings. These cravings can be decreased by eating more protein, keeping the body hydrated, consuming large amounts of healthy fats, and maintaining healthy bacteria in your gut. Also, when you do not eat sugar your blood sugar levels are more stable, and after a little while you will not crave sugar the way you did before.

Stop consuming sugar now. Say yes to a life with balanced blood sugar, stable moods, and no crash and burn after each meal.

Table sugar, sucrose, consists of two different sugar molecules, glucose and fructose. When consumed, sucrose is cleaved into glucose and fructose which are metabolized very differently by the body.

Glucose can be metabolized by every cell in the body and causes blood sugar raises, whereas fructose does not affect the blood sugar, and is only metabolized by the liver using a completely different pathway

Fructose is a simple sugar found in e.g. table sugar, high fructose corn syrup and fruit juice. We often think of fructose as a good form of sugar since it does not cause blood sugar issues. However, this way of thinking is not correct; there are other issues related to fructose.

Fructose has always been a part of our diet in small amounts, but the amounts present in a modern diet is very different than what you get from vegetables and fruits alone. We do tend to eat more and more fructose, both as a part of processed foods, sodas and store bought juices, but also from the ever-growing availability of (out of season, unripe) fruit. Below is some of the reasons you should beware of the amount of fructose you consume.

Fructose cannot be used directly as energy by the body's cells like glucose can. It is therefore metabolized in the liver, where it mostly is transformed into fat, and can cause fatty liver disease. Unfortunately, fructose can be toxic in high levels, and it damages the liver in the same way as alcohol. As mentioned in a very good documentary: Sugar The Bitter Truth:

"None of us would give our children alcohol, but juice all day long we do not think twice about!"

- It can decrease the binding of insulin to cells and therefore lead to insulin resistance.

- Fructose increase oxidative damage in our cells and contribute to inflammation when reacting with proteins and polyunsaturated fats forming advanced glycation end-products.

- Some people with digestive problems suffer from fructose malabsorption, and do not easily absorb fructose. It is therefore available for the bacteria in the gut and can create gut flora imbalances and promote overgrowth of pathogenic bacteria.

- Fructose can cause leptin resistance. Leptin is a hormone that is used to regulate appetite and to keep a normal metabolism.

- Cancer cells has shown to thrive very well on fructose as their energy source!

- During the metabolism of fructose, the bad cholesterol, VLDL, is formed in high amounts compared to the metabolism of glucose. We all want to avoid, VLDL, since it is associated with heart diseases.

From the above mentioned problems with fructose you might wonder how it is with fruit since it contains a lot of fructose. If you do not have fructose malabsorption there should be NO problems consuming ripe fruit in low to medium amounts (1-3 pieces a day). Fruits are not pure fructose, they are real foods with a low energy density, full of vitamins and with lots of fiber. It is hard to over-eat and you would need to eat an enormous amount to reach harmful levels of fructose. But when refined sugar (50% fructose) and High Fructose Corn Syrup (42% in foods and 55% in soda) is used, you get the free fructose with no added nutrition and no fiber, and in excess amounts the body cannot handle. Think twice when giving your kids a store bought juice and buy them an orange and a water bottle instead.

Processed foods

What are processed foods anyway? Processed foods are not found in nature, but are "foods" created in a complex laboratory to get the right taste, right texture and right package, to get the consumer to get addicted and buy the "food" again and again. Processed foods are often filled with artificial ingredients, sweeteners, sodium, preservatives and emulsifiers. So processed foods are not healthy because they:

- Often lack vitamins, minerals, protein and fiber. If vitamins are present, they are most likely artificial and added after processing.
- Are very often high in sugar and carbs.
- Are produced containing artificial ingredients, GMO substances, chemicals and preservatives.
- Contain high amounts of hydrogenated and partially-hydrogenated oils, which causes oxidative stress, inflammation and heart diseases.
- Are very often in plastic wrapping which can contain hormone disrupting chemicals.
- Are not high quality products. Most processed foods are made as cheap as possible with the food quality this entails.
- Have often been over-heated, ruining the nutrients.
- Contain artificial colors, some which have been linked to cancer and ADHD, like caramel color.
- Contain artificial flavoring. There are more than hundred laboratory chemicals designed to mimic natural flavors. Some research have suggested that artificial flavoring additives can

cause changes in human behavior.

Another issue with processed foods are the high amounts of processed salts. Not just any salt, because salt is an essential element of a healthy body, but processed salt striped from trace minerals and with added anti-caking additives. Many of the preservatives like ferrocyanide, magnesium carbonate, and aluminum hydroxide are not required to be listed on the containers, so the consumers do not even know what kind of bad chemicals they contain. Salt from natural sources contain up to 60 trace minerals, and are not processed in any way and therefore do not contain these toxic chemicals. Celtic Sea salt and Himalaya salt are two good choices of salt since they contain plenty of minerals that your body needs to function properly.

Canola oil is often advertised as a healthy oil, since it is high in polyunsaturated fat and contains very little amounts of saturated fat. Even though this is true, the problem with canola oil is the way it has been manufactured. Canola oil is a very processed oil, which has been exposed to high pressure, sodium hydroxide (lye) and bleach, all which leave you with a clean and odor free oil. The problem with the oil is that the polyunsaturated fat is not very stable, and the processing of canola oil forms large amounts of the harmful molecule, free radicals, which causes inflammation and harm the cells in the human body.

This also applies to other vegetable oils, like corn oil and soybean oil, which are also highly processed and contain the polyunsaturated fat that is very unstable under heat, light, solvents, and pressure.

When consuming oils high in free radicals it will activate your immune system and cause inflammation, damaging your cell membranes, contributing to heart disease, weight gain, and other degenerative diseases.

Grains

Removing grains for the diet is currently a very hot topic in the industry. It comes in a multitude of varieties like wheat, rye, rice, corn, quinoa, buckwheat, etc., and they are found in almost every standard meal across the globe. It has not always been like that, and there are many factors why I recommend removing all grains from your diet. At least for you to see how you feel without consuming them.

Increase blood sugar

Grains do raise our blood sugar, and especially process grains, and as discussed in the chapter about sugar, high blood sugar is not healthy for our bodies. Since almost every meal and every snack contain grains, our blood sugar will be like a roller-coaster just by the fact of eating grains. Grains will therefore leave you at some points with low blood sugar and no energy, afternoon dip after lunch where most people crave something sweet to keep going throughout the day.

Phytic acid

Another problem with grains is the content of phytic acid. Phytic acid binds to minerals and is located on the outer part of the grain. The reason it binds to these minerals is because when it gets out in the ground as a seed to make a new plant, it needs to hold on to all the nutrients so that this plant can thrive.

The Phytic acid does not only hold on to the nutrients that it has in itself, it also absorbs some of the nutrients that you eat at the same time. In other words, eating a mineral rich meal with rice, vegetables, protein, etc. will not give you all the minerals the meal contains. The grain Will actually absorb some of the minerals, which makes it unavailable for your body to obtain. Eating a lot of grains will rob your meals of these minerals, leading to possible mineral depletion. This will rob you of your energy and can leave you unhealthy and feeling tired, out of energy and fatigued.

We are always told to eat whole grains. I partly agree with that, but actually, in whole grains, there is much more phytic acid, which will make you have even less minerals available for your body. It is ironic that it is a common statement that grains are full of minerals when they actually deplete us. The minerals are not available for your body, so even though they are in the grain, your body cannot use them.

Lectins

The next thing on the list is lectins, of which the best-known is gluten. We have all heard about gluten allergy (celiac disease) and gluten sensitivity, and they are different aspects of the problems surrounding lectins. You can be gluten allergic where you cannot tolerate any at all and have an autoimmune disorder, or you can be gluten sensitive where the consequence of eating a little gluten is not as severe. With gluten sensitivity your immune system will not attack the gut wall as in gluten allergy, but can cause bloating, brain-fog and other unpleasant symptoms.

Lectin is a carbohydrate-binding protein, which means that it binds to sugar molecules. It is found in plants and animals, and in microbes and bacteria and it is a part of their defense mechanism.

Not all lectins are considered bad and some are very beneficial for us. Some of these beneficial lectins are found on a certain type of immune cells in the body and are a crucial part of our immune system in the defense against pathogens. The lectins bind to sugar molecules on the surface of bacteria and some viruses, including HIV, and helps the immune system identify the target. In this case, lectins are very beneficial in keeping us healthy and can help avoid serious infections to manifest. Unfortunately, the types of lectins that are found in grains do not serve this type of benefits, and are instead causing problems for our gut cells and immune system.

We humans cannot digest lectins, so they pass through our gut system as a whole molecule until something else can digest it. Unfortunately, lectins are a good source of food for the pathogenic bacteria in our gut, and if we feed the, they will increase in number. There is a threshold of how many pathogenic bacteria we can have in our system without them causing problems. When they increase in number, the chance of passing this threshold and having our daily lives affected increases. Pathogenic bacteria are a part of our ecosystem, but we do not want them to grow out of control.

Another issue with lectins from grains are that they bind to the cells of the gut lining or intestinal lining, where they make small gaps between the cells. This can cause leaky gut for some.

Leaky gut means that there is a possibility for the undigested food to transfer from the gut to the blood. We are not talking pieces of food, but food molecules that have yet to be broken down to a size the body can utilize outside of the intestines. These molecules can cause the immune system to react to food that is normally has no problem absorbing, but because the leaked food is not fully digested, it activates the immune system, causing inflammation. Some of the proteins that cross the gut lining and end up in the blood, have amino acid sequences that are identical to amino acid sequences on some human cells within our body. Because the immune system recognizes these undigested proteins as foreign it starts producing antibodies against the amino acid sequence. These antibodies flow around in the blood and recognize the same sequence at on human cells. Here it activates the immune system against our own body, causing an autoimmune disease. Depending on where our body has that unique amino acid sequence, the different types of autoimmune disorders occur.

The leaked molecules, which are perfectly normal in our gut, were never intended to be outside of the gut. Our body is not designed for having them in the blood stream, and they can cause headache, belly bloating, fatigue, inflammation. All these things are we do not want in our life and what makes us survive instead of thrive.

There are many different types of lectins in the different types of grain. Gluten is present in wheat and rye, but grains like rice and qinua contain other types of lectins. Some people are sensitive to all types of grains, whereas others are only sensitive to some of them. I want to highlight that not everyone is sensitive to lectins. Again, it is very important to use the Awareness Journal to understand if you are sensitive, so listen to your body and find out what is making you fatigued.

Another of the benefits of removing grains is a better digestion. When you have better digestion and have one-minute elimination, or you go to the restroom twice a day, you will easier remove the toxins that drain your body of energy. When you are constipated, the food can "rot" in your gut, slowly releasing toxins. Getting rid of the waste before toxins are released will give you elevated mood and tons of energy. Besides getting better digestion grains also increases the absorption of minerals, which are necessary to produce energy in your body.

The last thing I what to mention in regards to removing grains is that when you remove one item that causes inflammation and fatigue, you get one step closer to optimal health. I encourage you to think about what kind of benefit you think you might have from removing grain. We are different, and all have our "normal" quirks, which might not be so "normal" after all.

If you do want to reintroduce grains again, there is a couple of things you can do to remove or at least decrease phytic acid and lectins.

First of all, I encourage you to soak the grains in water overnight and rinse them before use. You can also ferment or sprout them, making it easier for you to digest. Fermenting lets bacteria and yeasts break down the phytic acid and lectins, whereas they are used and broken down by the plant during the spouting process.

Legumes, including soy and beans

Besides being high in carbohydrates and containing both phytic acid and lectins like grains, some legumes can contain phytoestrogens. Phyto meaning plant, so it is also called plant- estrogen.

Phytoestrogen is not really estrogen, but it acts like estrogen in the body, since it has the ability to bind to the same receptors as estrogen binds to. While the medical community has yet to fully cover and understand the biochemical pathways of phytoestrogens in the body, it is clear that phytoestrogens can cause hormonal unbalance.

Though eating legumes might not cause problems by itself, living in a world full of other environmental estrogens and hormone-disrupting chemicals, the hormonal disrupters just adds up. Legumes (especially soy) is an easy one to completely avoid.

Like grains, if you do decide to add in legumes to your diet, soaking, sprouting, cooking, and fermenting is always good in order to remove the anti-nutrients in these food. Add them in one at a time and pay attention to your Awareness Journal.

Dairy

Dairy is another food group that can cause problems for people. Some people do not tolerate lactose (milk sugar) very well, but some people do not even know that lactose might be their problem. These people are lactose intolerant and lack the enzymes necessary for proper break down and digestion of milk. As a result, they end up with bloating, diarrhea, and other digestion problems.

Other problems with dairy is the effect it has on the blood sugar, and that grain-fed cows produce milk with higher amounts of Omega-6 fatty acids and lower amounts of Omega-3 fatty acids compared to pastured cows. In the long-term, this can trigger chronic inflammation, and leave you feeling sick and energy depleted.

We have always been told that we need to consume dairy to keep our bones healthy and avoid fracture. Some of the latest research actually shows that the opposite is true. An increase in milk consumption has shown to increase the risk of bone fractures and in some cases also increase the risk of mortality from heart disease and cancer. Instead, you will get calcium from bone broth, nuts, seeds and cruciferous vegetables, such as kale, cabbage, broccoli and green leafy vegetables. Some research show that it is even easier for our body to absorb calcium from these sources compared to dairy, making them more available for our body to use.

Even though you tolerate lactose just fine, there are other issues with milk. Casein is a protein in milk that also causes problems for some people. Casein intolerance is not very known in the public, and most people think that if they are not lactose intolerant, then milk is not a problem for them. Unfortunately, that is not always the case, and especially people with digestive problems can have problems digesting this protein. As a result of mis-digestion of Casein, they end up with casomorhins which is highly addictive and affect the function of the brain negatively when absorbed though a damaged gut lining.

The only dairy products that I can recommend is grass-fed, pasture-raised and organic butter and ghee. Both are high in fat-soluble vitamins like vitamin A, E and K, contain Omega-3 fatty acids and butyrate which is anti-inflammatory and has powerful protective effects on the digestive system.

What to Eat

I have mentioned a lot of different food that should be avoided or at lease removed for a period of time to see if it helps on your energy levels. But if you remove, sugar, grains, dairy, legumes/beans and processed foods what is there left to actually eat?

Here is a list of the type of food that I encourage you to eat:

- Fresh or frozen vegetables
- Fresh fruits
- Wild caught or Organic farmed Fish/seafood
- Grass-fed meats (preferable organic)
- Eggs (preferable pasture-raised or organic)

- Nuts (excluding peanuts)

- Seeds

- Healthy fat and oil

If you want help to embrace this way of eating, I do offer some health coaching support, or you can have a look at my program A Life of THRIVE, which includes 14 days with suggested meals for breakfast, lunch and dinner. (www.AwesomeHealthy.Life/A-Life-of-THRIVE)

Eat a Rainbow of Vegetables and Fruit

What is it that all diets have in common? It does not matter if it is paleo, if it is low-fat, high- fat, vegan or raw. What they all have in common are vegetables.

All diets agree: Vegetables are good for you.

I really do encourage you to try to add one extra vegetable in every meal you have. If you are having Spaghetti Squash Bolognese, you already have squash and tomatoes in the dish, but try to add at least one extra vegetable to that meal as well. Whenever I cook, I have a standard recipe I follow for most dishes, and then I think, what can I do to add one more vegetable to this meal?

Often I make it really simple. I cut a cucumber, I make some carrot sticks or have some tomatoes on the side. I just have them raw because that is really simple and easy.

"Always try to add in one extra vegetable and aim for a rainbow of colors each day!"

We have all heard it: "You need to have a balanced diet", but really what does it mean, and how do we do that? I encourage you to try this simple approach. Eat a rainbow of vegetables and fruit! By eating all the colors of the rainbow everyday your body will get all the vitamins, minerals, fibers and a lot of other nutrients like phytonutrients that the body needs to be healthy!

Phytonutrients (also referred to as phytochemicals) are compounds, which serve various functions in the plants, helping to protect its vitality. Some phytonutrients protect the plant from insect attack while others protect against UV radiation.

Fruits and vegetables are concentrated sources of phytonutrients compared to other types of foods. Since many phytonutrients also serve as the pigment that gives foods their colors, you can absorb many phytonutrients by eating a plate full of colorful vegetables and fruits. As we eat the rainbow of colors, we absorb all the different phytonutrients present in each color, and use their defense mechanisms to help our bodies function better. These phytonutrients are the anti-inflammatory, detoxifying, anti-oxidant and hormone-balancing compounds that we should eat every day to prevent disease and create optimal health!

THEREFORE, AIM FOR A RAINBOW OF COLORS EVERYDAY!

On the picture below, I have shared some ideas for you to get inspired to try new fruit and vegetables. Look at this chart before going grocery shopping and get inspired to try something new this week!

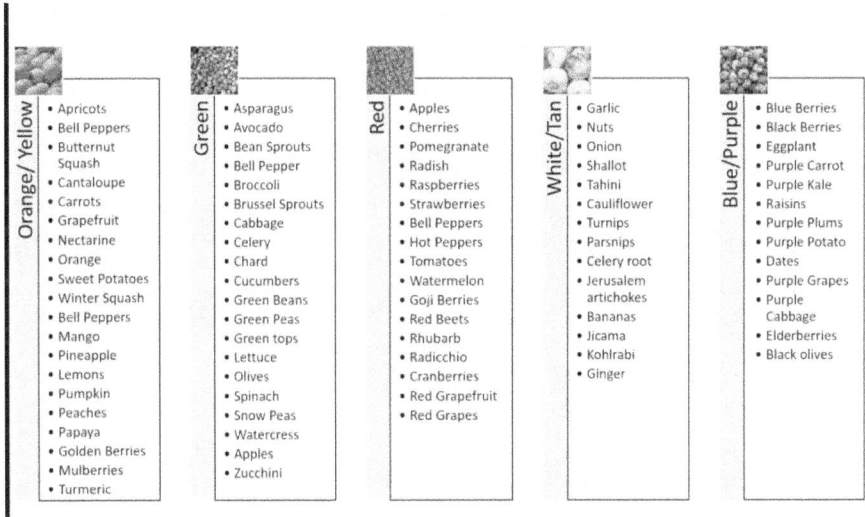

Orange/Yellow	Green	Red	White/Tan	Blue/Purple
• Apricots	• Asparagus	• Apples	• Garlic	• Blue Berries
• Bell Peppers	• Avocado	• Cherries	• Nuts	• Black Berries
• Butternut Squash	• Bean Sprouts	• Pomegranate	• Onion	• Eggplant
• Cantaloupe	• Bell Pepper	• Radish	• Shallot	• Purple Carrot
• Carrots	• Broccoli	• Raspberries	• Cauliflower	• Purple Kale
• Grapefruit	• Brussel Sprouts	• Strawberries	• Turnips	• Raisins
• Nectarine	• Cabbage	• Bell Peppers	• Parsnips	• Purple Plums
• Orange	• Celery	• Hot Peppers	• Celery root	• Purple Potato
• Sweet Potatoes	• Chard	• Tomatoes	• Jerusalem artichokes	• Dates
• Winter Squash	• Cucumbers	• Watermelon	• Bananas	• Purple Grapes
• Bell Peppers	• Green Beans	• Goji Berries	• Jicama	• Purple Cabbage
• Mango	• Green Peas	• Red Beets	• Kohlrabi	• Elderberries
• Pineapple	• Green tops	• Rhubarb	• Ginger	• Black olives
• Lemons	• Lettuce	• Radicchio		
• Pumpkin	• Olives	• Cranberries		
• Peaches	• Spinach	• Red Grapefruit		
• Papaya	• Snow Peas	• Red Grapes		
• Golden Berries	• Watercress			
• Mulberries	• Apples			
• Turmeric	• Zucchini			

Please do try to eat a variety of different vegetables and fruits within the same color since a carrot and an orange bell pepper do not necessarily have the same phytonutrients.

"Less than 50% of adults consume daily the recommended fruit and vegetables."

When I say eating the rainbow, it is not only having one vegetable from each group, but try to eat a balanced diet where you try different fruits and vegetable in the same group each week. This way you get the benefits of all the different phytonutrients that are present in the different fruit and vegetables.

Step #3: Life Balance for Endless Energy

I want to introduce you to a fun exercise that I want you to do every three months. It will give you an idea of which areas of your life that you need to work on in order to have Life Balance for Endless Energy.

It does not matter how much healthy food you eat, and how much sugar you avoid, you will be left drained of energy if you are very stressed or if you have a job that gives absolutely no joy. Our lives need to be in balance to create a life full of energy and joy.

Take a look at the chart below and simply follow the instructions below.

Wheel of Balance

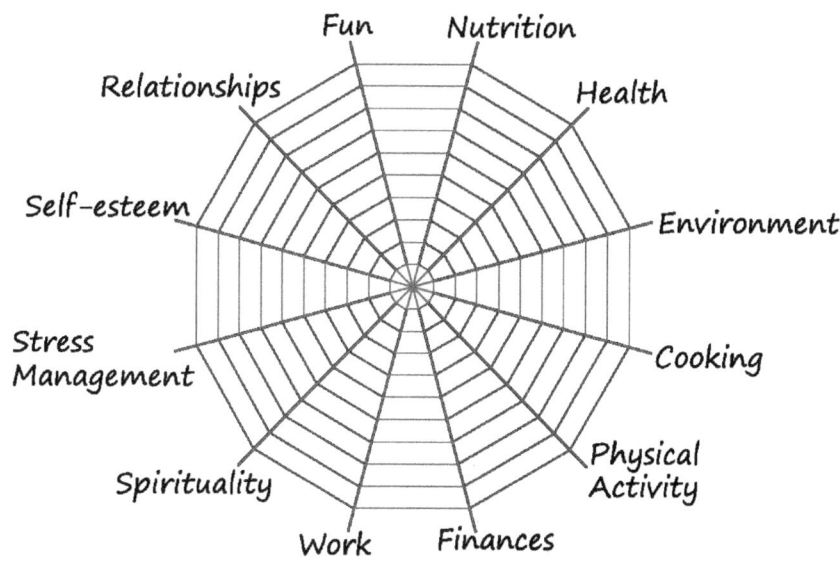

How to Use the Life Balance for Endless Energy:

1. Place a dot on the line within each category to represent how your current status is.

2. The center indicate you are not satisfied with the situation and the outer indicate you are extremely happy about how things are.

3. Connect the dots with a line and see how your Life Balance looks like.

4. Which areas of your life are you scoring really low in? These are the areas you should have focus on the next three months in order to achieve a Life Balance for Endless Energy.

How does it look for you? Are you having a balanced life or is it clear for you which areas you need to work on in order to feel more balanced and increase your energy?

Chose one or two categories that you want to be working on the next three months. Find out which simple things you can do each week to move the dot for these categories closer to the edge of the circle. If you are low in fun, brainstorm on things you think is fun to do and leave you with energy. Commit on doing one of these things every week for the next three months in order for you to get more balanced.

Repeat the exercise again after three months and see how it has changed. Did you manage to lift the two categories that you scored low on? How does it look now, and which categories do you choose to have focus on for the next three months?

Step #4: Gut Health for Endless Energy

When we eat, we are exposed to bacteria, viruses and toxins through the food, and our body has a unique and successful system to make sure we are affected as little as possible. Most of us know this as the immune system, but there is another, crucial part of this protection that most people are completely unaware of. It is a symbiosis known as the gut flora, and it consist of an intricate, balanced mix of different microbes. The number of bacteria in our bodies outnumbers human cells 10:1.

The gut flora consists of both beneficial bacteria and yeast, and some of their functions are:

- Culture the gut lining making no room for pathogens.
- Making sure pathogenic bacteria, pathogenic yeast and viruses does not harm the body.
- Bind to toxins and leave the body holding on to the toxins.
- Produce vitamins that are vital for our bodies, like B vitamins and vitamin K.
- Help with digestion of foods that the stomach acid and digestion enzymes have not been able to digest.

Gut health is an extremely important aspect of overall health. Many, if not all, gut related conditions are affected by what we eat. Research show that imbalance in the gut flora is linked to all kinds of diseases like Alzheimer, Cancer, Autism, ADHD, Depression, Autoimmunity, Allergies and much more.

Hippocrates said it best: "All disease begins in the gut."

One key issue for a healthy gut and a healthy gut lining is to maintain beneficial bacteria in the gut. However, with the society we have today, many people do not have the variety of species, and the amount of beneficial bacteria that are needed for optimal health. Most people today have been on antibiotics several times in their life, have taken birth control pills and are consuming foods containing pesticides or other harmful chemicals which all kill our small friends in our digestive system. When the good and beneficial bacteria are killed, it leaves space on the gut wall for pathogenic bacteria to grow, and it can take from months to years to restore. In some cases, if nothing is actively done, it will never recover.

Some problems with having pathogenic bacteria culturing the gut lining are that they can interfere with the gut cells and cause leaky gut. The pathogenic bacteria also produce toxins which can be transported into the blood stream and affect the health of your body. Furthermore, because the gut wall cells are relying on healthy bacteria to give them 60-70% of their energy, the pathogenic bacteria will leave the gut wall cells malnourished when they have replaced the beneficial bacteria. With malnourished cells in the gut wall, the cells are not able to maintain their normal functions. This leads to an inability to digest and absorb nutrients, malabsorption, nutritional deficiencies and food intolerances.

As I have mention earlier in the book, to empty your bowl every day is very important for optimal health and energy. I have therefore included some ideas of how to remove and prevent constipation:

Lemon water

A big glass as the first thing in the morning, also try adding in some apple cider vinegar.

Carrot juice

Try starting the morning with a glass of fresh homemade carrot juice.

Wash the carrots and leave the skin on if it looks okay. The bacteria from the soil is good for your gut flora balance.

Flax seed meal

A can of coconut milk, ¼ cup of (grinded) flaxseeds and half a banana blended and stored in fridge overnight.

Probiotic

Each morning, as well as cultured foods and beverages.

Flax oil

1 teaspoon per day can be taken if you do not consume grinded flaxseeds. You can add it to a salad, smoothie or alone.

Magnesium citrate

200-400 mg when needed. Personally, I only use this if above does not work, and I start with 200 mg before going to bed. If it does not help the morning, I would take 200 mg more. Remember to drink a lot of water as well.

One thing is to get rid of your waste, another thing is to restore and maintain a healthy gut. Here are some suggestions of how to do that:

- Make sure you have proper elimination 1-2 times a day.

- Take probiotics every day.

- Add in cultured foods like sauerkraut, kimchi, raw yogurt and raw kefir (if dairy is tolerated).

- Add in cultured beverages like water and coconut kefir, kombucha.

- Avoid taking antibiotics whenever possible, they do not only kill the bad bacteria but also the good ones.

- If taking antibiotics, ask the doctor to give you narrow spectrum antibiotics, since it is not killing as many beneficial bacteria compared to wide spectrum antibiotics.

- Remember that antibiotics do not help against influenza and other viruses.

- Avoid the problematic foods mentions in the chapter Food for Endless Energy.

- De-stress.

When starting on probiotics it is very important to start slowly. When you add extra, beneficial bacteria into your system, they will kill some of the pathogenic ones. When they die, their cell wall will be disrupted (apoptosis) and the toxic substances inside the bacteria will be released into the intestine lumen, and some of the toxins will be absorbed into the body. If taking a huge amount of probiotics at once, you can get a die-off. Die-off is any type of effect caused by the toxins released when the pathogenic bacteria dies by apoptosis. Symptoms of die-off can be anything from headache to eczema and even flu-like symptoms and muscle and joint pain. The amount of die-off you experience depends on the proportion of pathogenic bacteria in your gut flora, and the amount of probiotic you take. I therefore recommend that you start with a very low dose of probiotic and slowly increase it over time. If you do experience die- off, cut down the amount of probiotic and go even slower. Do not stop taking the probiotic, since we want to have those pathogenic bacteria killed and so you can create room for more beneficial bacteria in the gut.

Some people have very severe gut health problems, and though they will benefit by following These 6 Steps, I highly recommend trying the GAPS diet by Dr. Natasha Campbell-McBride. If you are interested in learning more about the possibilities to heal your gut problems with the GAPS Diet, please do not hesitate to contact me.

On a final note, I implore you to remember that:

If you keep your gut healthy, it will also keep you healthy!

Step #5: Evening Routines for Endless Energy

You ask why the evening routines are so important that they need their own step. Evening routines are something that we do not give very much attention in our modern world, but it can be a key factor in order to get your life into balance and increase energy.

How you spend the last few hours before bedtime is essential in the quality and quantity of your sleep, and how easy you fall asleep and wake up. Sleep is not just something we need in order to have energy the next morning. Sleep is essential for all vital functions of your body, and many critical bodily activities occur during sleep. Some of the activities are processing of memories and release of hormones controlling stress, appetite and metabolism. To work optimally, these activities need quality sleep, preferably for 7-9 hours every night. If you make this a habit, your body will in return give you increased energy and focus, a stronger immune system, better overall mood and less stress.

If you use excess amount of time and energy thinking about something specific right before bedtime, most of us have experienced having dreams or nightmares about that specific thing. It is therefore a bad idea to watch or read something that upsets you, or make your head wander, right before you go to sleep. Instead, try to calm down your mind by focusing on de- stressing and doing something pleasant for yourself prior to going to bed.

Here are some suggestions that you can do in the evening in order to get better sleep at night:

- Do not eat after 8 pm.
- Turn off TV, computer or other stimuli with intense light 2 hours before bedtime.
- Dim the lights to produce more melatonin.
- Listen to relaxing music or meditate.
- Take a hot bath with Epsom salts before bed.

- Make a list of all the things you are grateful for.

- Go to bed by 10 pm and follow the daylight cycle if possible.

Melatonin is a hormone in the body that regulates your sleep-wake cycle. This hormone is regulated by light exposure, so the more light you get during the evening, the lower levels of melatonin your body will produce, and you will be more awake. Higher levels melatonin can be created by diming the light and turning of TV, computers and iPads before bedtime. This will leave you more tired and give you a deeper and better quality of sleep.

Another issue that is very common in our society is to take an evening snack after 8 pm and close to bedtime. This leaves your body with no other alternative than to focus on digesting the food you consumed, and it is forced to postpone other important activities that normally happens during sleep, such as processing of memories and release of hormones controlling stress, appetite and metabolism.

Step #6: Positive Mindset for Endless Energy

As you have learned in Step #3: Life Balance for Endless Energy, it is not only food that gives us energy, it is all aspects of our lives.

One of the very important things that has a profound impact on our quality of life, health and happiness, and therefore also our energy level, is the way we think and our thinking patterns.

If you have not thought about this before, you might think it is a little weird and unnatural to have focus on your thoughts.

But really, what are your thoughts throughout your day, your week and your life? Your thoughts can either be happy and supportive or negative and destructive, or maybe even a mixture of both. In that case, be aware of the elements of your life in which you are thinking negative, and what situations triggers it.

Negative and destructive thinking patterns could go something like this: I wish I did not have to go to work today, I just know that it will be stressful as always! Typical me, I forgot my car keys in the apartment, why do I always forget them? Up the stairs one more time. How can it be that there is NEVER a parking spot, and I need to walk 10 minutes to get to work, and this makes me late again!

A person with positive and supportive thinking patterns could go something like this: I am so glad I woke up 5 minutes before my alarm clock, I feel fully energized for a new day at work! I know we have a lot to do, but I am glad that I am being challenged and can show my boss my full potential! Ups, I forgot my car keys in the apartment again today – more good exercise for me. I always have trouble finding a parking spot in front of the work building, I will just park at the first available one down the road. That is more exercise for me and I will not be as late as if I started searching for one that was closer. Anyway, no one ever notices that I am late anyway, and I will just stay 5 minutes more at the end of the day.

This can be the one and same person, and you can make that shift of having a more positive approach to life.

Research shows that a person who focuses on the negative will have a lower quality of life, burn out much quicker and be sicker compared to a person choosing to focus on the positive aspects of the same situations.

We have all heard about the placebo effect, which is the effect of getting cured by believing in the treatment, rather than by the drug itself. The opposite effect has also been shown to be true. If you believe that something will make you sick, the thoughts alone can have that effect. This phenomenon is called the nocebo effect, and will occur when people see the negative aspects of life and always focus on that.

People tend to say that it is easy to focus on the positive for some and not for others, but that is really not true. It is only a matter of how willing you are to change your life and your thoughts! We humans tend to hold on to our negative thoughts and identify them as being a part of who we are, but they are not!

We allow them to take over our life, because we are thought to do this.

So how do we change this negative, downward going spiral to a positive upward going spiral? First of all, it is really simple and I have done it myself, but you need to be persistent!

I grew up the same way many other people do, learning to find the five mistakes. Literally this is an exercise in school or kids drawing books. Two almost identical pictures are shown next to each other, and you need to find the five mistakes!

My life turned out like most others; I found the mistakes in my own life and focused on them with all my energy. Everyone in school is better than me, I cannot read as fast as the others can, I am not as skinny as that girl, why am I not the most popular girl in the class? Why is my nose so big? This negative and destructive thinking pattern has followed me for years, or to be exact, until I was 30 years old! Imagine how much destruction that can do on your self- esteem and self-worth, and then adding on that I was not feeling very well;

I felt like I was failing in every aspect of my life!

During the period of my life where I decided to unplug and only focus on my healing, I found that people that had recovered from the same symptoms as I had, both changed their diet, but also changed their thoughts for more positive ones. I had nothing to lose and decided it was worth trying!

"A thought is only a thought, and a thought can be changed!"
by Louise Hay

Here are a few simple things you can do to change your thoughts:

a. Every evening before falling asleep think about at least five things you are grateful for.

b. Write a positive sentence about yourself on the mirror so it is the first thing you see in the morning and the last thing you see at night, e.g. "I am worth loving!", "I love myself" or "I am always doing my best!".

c. If you have a negative experience that keeps going through your head, write it down and tear the paper apart. Rewrite the story the way you actually want it to be, with lots of positive words and emotions!

d. When you become aware of a negative thought, tell your thought, "I am letting you go, you do not deserve my attention anymore. I replace this emotion with happiness, love and balance."

e. Find a song that makes you happy, and sing it out load! I know it sounds silly, but it really works! I can be really sad and irritated, and whenever I sing a certain song from my childhood, my mood can totally shift. I sing it loader and loader until I am able to sing it with passion and happiness in my voice! It goes something like this:

"Today I am so happy, so happy, so happy, everything's fantastic,

and the life is wonderful!"

Another silly song that can raise my mood is the one from the Lego® song "Everything is Awesome"

f. Use this breathing exercise by Dr. Andrew Weil to calm you down and reduce the stressful thoughts. I actually use it every night before falling asleep. http://www.drweil.com/drw/u/VDR00112/The-4-7-8-Breath-Benefits-and- Demonstration.html

g. These affirmations by Louise Hay, make you focus on the positive things already present in your life. https://youtu.be/tsgoG2UrxVM

h. Meditation is a good way to calm your mind and reduce a negative thinking.

i. Try this guided meditation before sleeping by Glenn Harrold - Relax and sleep well,https://itunes.apple.com/us/app/relax-sleep-well-by- glenn/id412690467?mt=8 or this guided meditation by Vishen Lakhiani to let go of burdens and set an intention for the future, http://youtu.be/EaRu14P9H84.

j. Emotional Freedom Technique (EFT) is a method that can be used to reduce or remove stress, anxiety and even pain, even though you do not believe in it. Read more about EFT here: (http://www.thetappingsolution.com/).

You can try a session by listening to this video by Brad Yates and just simply follow his instructions. This is a video about how to let go of negative thinking and expecting the best. https://www.youtube.com/watch?v=NgyC318_wX0

Client Success Stories

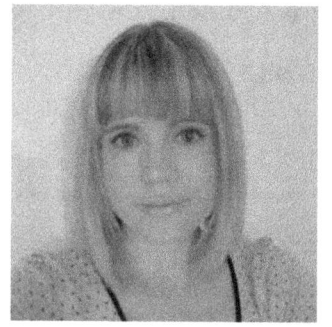

When I started working with Linda, my top three goals were to increase energy, get healthy, and enjoy life some more. Linda opened my eyes to healthy living by being educating and supporting in every step of the way!

During the 6 months I have had Linda as my Health Coach, I have not only gotten healthier, I have also gotten more confident, and I am now present in every moment of my life. I have learned not to chase someone else's expectations or dreams and instead be mindful about the important things in my own life. When I wake up today, I do so more energized and with a positive mindset, ready for the new day. I feel much more balanced and my quality of life has improved radically. Linda is an extremely dedicated and hard-working Health Coach, which takes the client on with her whole heart! If you put forth the effort to want a change you will surely have a strong, supportive and knowledgeable ally at your side that is eager to help YOU reach YOUR goals. I can tell you from my own experience that if you team up with Linda as your Health Coach, it will change your life for the better!

Íris Björg Bergmann Þorvaldsdóttir, 31 years old, Copenhagen

www.ammekonsulenterne.dk

Having a desk job and a lifestyle that does not include a lot of exercise, I found myself going down a spiral of unhealthy decisions. I contacted Linda knowing that I had do try and do something about it.

I was very skeptical about what she would be able to do. I figured she would tell me to eat less, only eat veggies and go exercise for 1 hour every day. This was not the case however. Linda introduced me to paleo and after some researching on my own I decided to give it a try. Linda was a great support throughout the transition process and helped with recipes and mental support to get through.

Five months in I find myself feeling great. I have more energy, a more positive attitude and a passion for life than I cannot remember having, ever. I used to wake up at 9 am feeling like I could easily sleep for 3 more hours. Now I wake up at 7 am, jump out of bed and are fully rested.

Linda has given me the tools I need to maintain this new lifestyle for the long run. Looking back today, contacting Linda was the best thing I could have done and I am happy to give her my warm felt recommendation.

Frank, 31 years old, Copenhagen

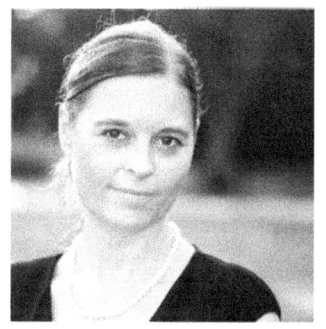

When I first met Linda, she came across as very knowledgeable on healthy food and introduced me to the paleo diet. Not only was she knowledgeable, she gained the knowledge by getting her own body on the right course, so it immediately became clear that this was not all theory.

As I had educated myself about how to avoid toxins in my body and had always been very interested in healthy food, I realized that

Linda could take me an extra step. So I decided to take one of her free coaching sessions after which I was convinced that I could not afford not to invest in the future health of my body, so I decided to sign up for Linda's 6 months program.

I gave the paleo diet a shot and the first week I lost 6 pounds but what was even better; I had more energy (did not get that energy dip in the afternoon that made me go and get that 2nd coffee) and my mood was much better.

I will be completely honest, changing your life to a healthy life is not easy. A health coach is there to guide and support you, but you have to do all the hard work. So it requires dedication and determination.

I used to say my eye surgery was the best investment I ever did, however signing up with Linda definitely competes with that.

Peggy Høegh, 39 years old, Houston

Blog Posts for Endless Energy

Do Not Fall Into the Holes...

Poem by Portia Nelson

"I walk down the street. There is a deep hole in the sidewalk.

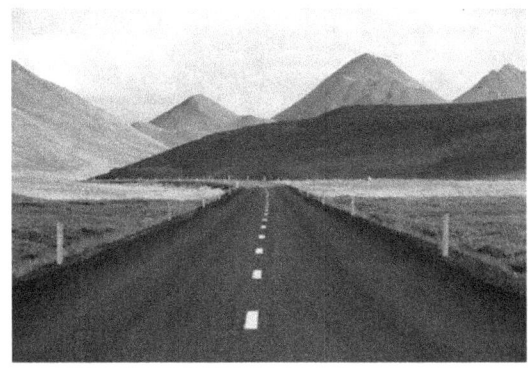

I fall in.

I am lost... I am helpless. It isn't my fault.

It takes forever to find a way out.

I walk down the same street. There is a deep hole in the sidewalk.

I pretend I don't see it. I fall in again.

I can't believe I am in the same place. But, it isn't my fault.

It still takes me a long time to get out.

I walk down the same street.

There is a deep hole in the sidewalk. I see it is there.

I still fall in. It's a habit. My eyes are open.

I know where I am.

It is my fault. I get out immediately.

walk down the same street.

There is a deep hole in the sidewalk. I walk around it.

I walk down another street."

— Portia Nelson, *There's a Hole in My Sidewalk: The Romance of Self-Discovery*

I came across this poem today, when writing an email to a client... I have heard it before and the first time I read it, it really hit me... I was doing exactly that, falling down the same hole again and again...

The hole of not feeling good enough, and talking myself down - to the point of stress.

I realized I needed to change! I needed to believe in myself and not focus on the holes! There will always be holes, everywhere we go in life! But we can choose not to focus on them and focus on the part of the road that is actually fully perfect!!

To be honest with you, there is actually more perfect roads out there than there is hole, so why focus on them at all!! It is like when you are driving a car in the dark and there is a tree along the road, if you focus too much on the tree you will drive into it, and smash the car. We all know that so we become aware of the tree but focus on the road!!

I want you to live your life like that! Be aware of the holes in the road, but keep focus on the perfect road in front of you!!! Do not be scared of the holes that might show up in the future - focus on what is NOW and what is right in front of you. Take one step at a time steering perfectly around the holes and keeping you on the perfect road!

THE ROAD TO HEALTH, HAPPINESS AND JOY IS RIGHT IN FRONT OF YOU - IT IS YOUR CHOICE!

STAY ON THE ROAD!

Fake It till You Become IT!

A friend of mine introduced me to this TED talk with Amy Cuddy: Your body language shapes who you are.

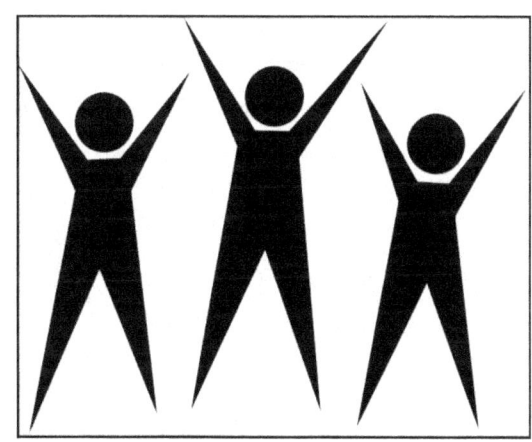

I had heard about it before; that your posture will not only effect how other people see you but also how you see and feel about yourself.

In this video Amy Cuddy shares the scientific data about how we by using power poses for 2 minutes can

affect the testosterone and the cortisol levels in the brain. By doing this we can reduce our stress levels and become more confident.

Watch the TED talk now: https://youtu.be/Ks- Mh1QhMc

This can be very beneficial in our daily life, maybe you have a job interview or any type of situation where you feel little nervous. Try it, stand up straight, lift your head high and put your arms on the sides of your hips, stand like that for 2 minutes and see what happens.

I know that it can feel fake and uncomfortable to stand with power when you really feel small and want to hide, but I promise you that if you really do try it, it works! You will feel less stressed, more confident and even happier. As Amy says - "Fake it till you become it!"

In what way can you see this being beneficial in your life?

The Best Gluten Free and Dairy Free Bread I have Ever Tasted!

Since I cannot tolerate any type of grains, I have tried making a lot of different types of bread, and this one is our absolute favorite!

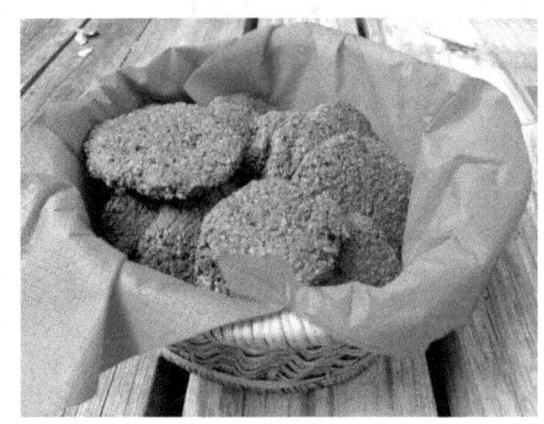

So if you want to cut down on wheat, or just want to try a healthy bread - try out this fabulous recipe!

Ingredients:

- 100 g (3.5 oz.) Flax seed
- 100 g (3.5 oz.) Shredded coconut or 50g coconut flour 100 g (3.5 oz.) Pumpkin seeds
- 200 g (7 oz.) Carrot pulp from homemade carrot juice or 100 g (3.5 oz.) almonds 6 Eggs
- 6 tbsp. Red palm oil or coconut oil
- Small amount of Sea salt or Himalaya salt 1 tsp. Baking soda
- 2 tbsp. Apple cider vinegar

Procedure:

Preheat the oven to 150° C or 300° F.

All ingredients except apple cider vinegar is placed in a food processor and mixed until the mass is even.

You can also just mix in a bowl if whole nuts are not used.) Add in Apple cider vinegar and mix well.

Form the bread buns on a flat oven rack covered with parchment paper. They can be a bit sticky, but do your best to make them round. Bake in the middle of the oven at for 35-40 minutes.

If you do not have a juicer you can always exchange the juice pulp with 150 g (3.5 oz.) ground almonds!

All seeds can be changed to whatever seeds and nuts you have in your cupboard! My bread buns are never the same. Try sesame seeds, chia seeds, cashew nuts, almonds, sunflower seeds and so on! There are so many possibilities!

This is the best gluten free and dairy free bread I have ever tasted! And they are even 100% without grains.

Delicious Egg Muffins

Whether you are looking for a new breakfast recipe, need a healthy toddler lunch or just want something you can grab as a healthy snack - these delicious egg muffins is a great choice!

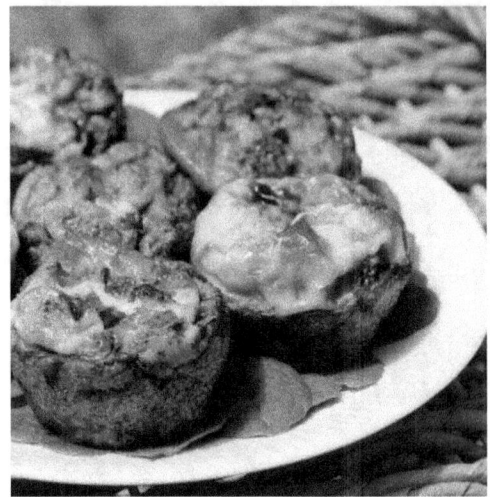

Ingredients:

- 2 cups Spinach, fresh or frozen 2 cups Broccoli, fresh or frozen 6 Eggs
- Sea salt or Himalaya salt Pepper

Procedure:

Turn on the oven at 400° F or 200° C Whip the eggs

Season with salt and pepper

Place spinach and broccoli in the muffin forms (I use a hard metal form for 12 muffins) Poor in the whipped eggs

Place the muffin plate in the middle of the oven and bake of 20 minutes.

We absolutely love these egg muffins; it is an easy way to get both some good protein as well as the benefits more vegetables. You can always try these muffins with different types of vegetables, or maybe add in some bacon for an extra flavor. Try out different vegetables and find your own favorite taste.

www.ingramcontent.com/pod-product-compliance
Lightning Source LLC
Chambersburg PA
CBHW071120280526
45787CB00003B/1104